FIT
PREGNANCY
& BEYOND

Your fit pregnancy
- & -
Post baby shape up guide

AMELIA RICCI

Qualified Pre & Postnatal Fitness Professional

FIT Pregnancy & Beyond
Your fit pregnancy & Post baby shape up guide
Amelia Ricci, Qualified Pre & Postnatal Fitness Professional

First Edition

Print Book ISBN 978-0-6482458-1-0
e-Book ISBN 978-0-6482458-0-3

Interior layout design by Mariana Vidakovics De Victor

www.livingbeautyfitness.com

You Tube: Amelia Ricci 4 week bikini body fitness

Facebook: AmeliaRicciSportsModelFitnessTrainer

Instagram: @livingbeautyamelia

CONTENTS

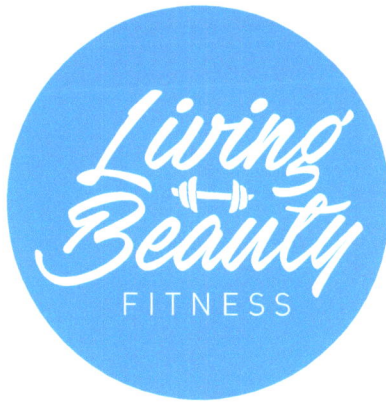

FIT PREGNANCY & BEYOND

There are many benefits to be gained from regular exercise during pregnancy. These include physical benefits and the prevention of excessive weight gain, as well as benefits for psychological wellbeing.

In addition to pregnancy-specific benefits, there are significant life-long benefits of regular exercise for all adults including reduced risk of cardiovascular disease, type 2 diabetes and some cancers.

Before you start an exercise program during your pregnancy, speak with your doctor or midwife to make sure that you do not have any health issues that may prevent you from participating in regular exercise during your pregnancy.

If there are no health or pregnancy reasons why you should not exercise, you should be encouraged during your pregnancy to participate in regular aerobic and strengthening exercises.

ABOUT AMELIA RICCI
& YOUR FIT PREGNANCY AND POSTNATAL JOURNEY

If you're reading FIT Pregnancy I know you love all things fitness and want to learn what is safe for your baby and yourself during this special time. Your body and mind will go through many changes during pregnancy and it is important to understand the current guidelines on safe exercise during pregnancy, so you can follow guidelines and modify your routine accordingly. In this guide we will examine exactly what you can expect including changes in weight, skeletal and muscle structure, but also the important mental and emotional side of pregnancy so you can have a journey that is safe but also enjoyable!

This guide will also give you the exercises to strengthen and rehabilitate your core muscles to begin to build back up to health and fitness after your beautiful baby is born. This important part of a mother's journey is often overlooked in the first few months after baby is born, but it doesn't have to take away precious time or energy. The exercises provided in Amelia's postnatal guide can be done in as little as 10 minutes per day at home.

ABOUT AMELIA

Amelia is Coach and Owner of Living Beauty Fitness. Qualified Pre and Postnatal Pilates Instructor, Yoga Teacher, Les Mills Instructor and Personal Trainer, Certified with Fitness Australia for over 15 years.

"I started out enjoying training at the gym as a stress relief from University studies, and then progressed to competing as a Fitness Model, winning 2 x Overall Sports Model Titles with ICN (iCompete Natural). Now I'm a mum to Orlando who is a very active 3-year-old boy and I'm also currently pregnant with my second baby!"

"I train girls to achieve their dreams as Fitness and Bikini Models. I also have a passion for safe and effective pre and postnatal exercise as I have specialised in Personal Training, Pilates and Yoga for pregnancy for many years, but I found it very challenging when I became pregnant! I realised the challenges that you face during pregnancy first hand, and now I can relate, going through two pregnancies."

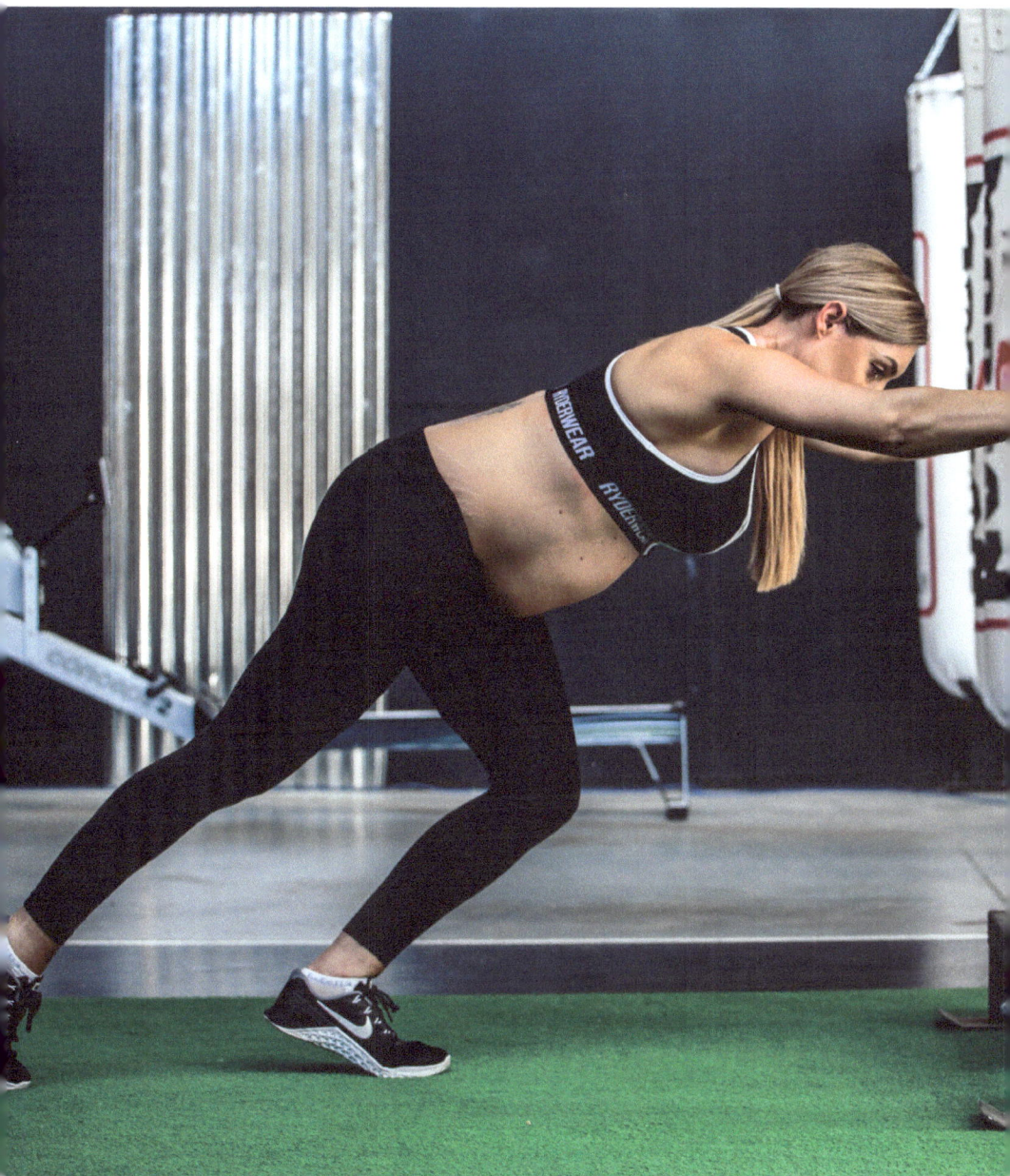

CHANGES I EXPERIENCED DURING MY PREGNANCIES
(PHYSICALLY, PSYCHOLOGICALLY AND EMOTIONALLY)

I am not one of those women who find it easy, pregnancy is hard, and you need support, during the pregnancy and especially when the baby is born. Emotionally it can be very difficult to accept the changes in your body, particularly the weight gain, exhaustion and the inability to exercise at a high intensity. Physically I have experienced back and hip pain, but I learned that this is all normal and is preparing the body to soften and expand to accommodate a growing baby. Once you have been through one pregnancy it is easier to comprehend that the level of joy at the end of your journey is so great, everything is worth it!

A new baby brings so much joy and happiness, but the responsibilities can also be a juggling act. Many people overlook the challenges faced as a mother of a newborn and the first six to twelve months can be extremely demanding with the routine of feeding, settling and trying to establish sleep for the baby and the parents. You will likely have some good weeks and other weeks are like climbing a mountain and never feeling like you will reach the end of the journey. Babies cry on average for 6-8 hours each day and this is emotionally draining, as quite often as parents we put in 120% effort, but feel like our baby is still not happy. Hang in there, you will get through the challenges and help is available at your local Family Health Service or Doctor. Reach out for help rather than trying to struggle through the days and nights!

HOW QUICKLY CAN YOU BOUNCE BACK FROM PREGNANCY?

Post pregnancy with Orlando I had to recover from an emergency caesarean which was hard because not only was my pelvic floor weakened from hours of pushing, we eventually had to resort to a c section and therefore the ab muscles are cut, and this is major internal surgery. During my labour Orlando got stuck the wrong way and during every contraction his heart rate plummeted, which meant my birth plan went out the window and we were rushed into surgery for an unplanned c section. Many women forget it is not just the external scar, there is also a lot of internal stitching that needs to heal.

I learned a lot from my first pregnancy and listened to exactly what I was told in terms of avoiding any exercise for 6 weeks. Even though I have studied and taught pregnancy fitness for years, nothing prepared me for how confronting it was emotionally to recover from the birth. It did get better and each week I saw a physio for exercises and I never did any impact work or heavier weights until my core was strong again and I was cleared by my medical practitioner.

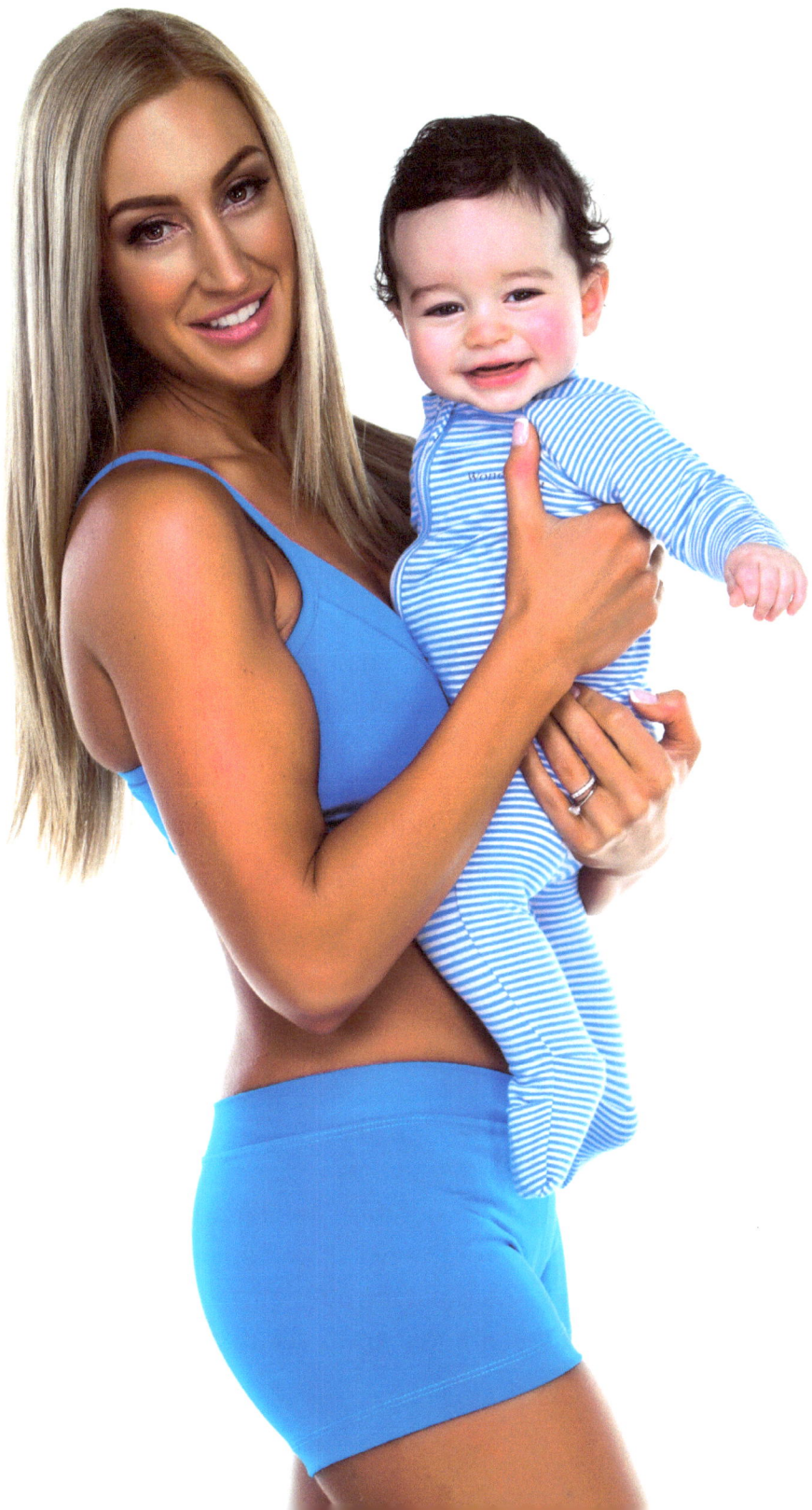

I gained 25 kilos during my first pregnancy and lost all the baby weight to compete in my best condition in a bikini model comp, 12 months later. So, my message for new mama's is not to worry, it is certainly possible to get your strength back, get flat abs and achieve whatever you desire you just need to follow advice, do Pilates exercises prescribed by a professional and be consistent and patient.

It can be hard not to compare yourself to photos on social media, but it's a case of only 1% of the population of women that bounce back super-fast. Most women I have trained (over 15 years' experience) simply do not bounce back, and you must remember that those Instagram babes that have a flat tummy two weeks later are the minority.

Every woman carries their baby differently and it depends on your unique body structure including height, how long your torso is and how many children you have had and what your previous pregnancies were like. Comparison as they say is the thief of joy, so I encourage all new mothers to embrace the journey, eat some chocolate or whatever you enjoy and if you are staying active and eating healthy most of the time, don't stress about weight gain. You will get your body back and this is the most incredible and empowering journey the last thing you want to do is stress out and worry about how fast you get your body back.

HOW MY TRAINING CHANGED DURING PREGNANCY

I think there's a misconception that you need to train daily during pregnancy. Even 3-4 days a week is beneficial and focusing on muscles such as back (for posture), legs (specifically glutes) as they are a key stabiliser for the pelvis and spine. It's important to also train your arms to maintain the strength needed to lift baby, plus bend over the cot and lifting a pram in and out of the car!

There are so many variations to weights exercises that can be done safely and the main modifications I incorporate are:

* Eliminate abs and inner thigh exercises as these muscles need to loosen to accommodate your growing baby.

* Reduce and gradually stop impact work, especially in the second and third trimester jumping and plyo should be ceased due to the hormones acting to softening joints and increasing the risk of injury. It can also be very uncomfortable jumping when boobs and tummy are large!

FEAR ASSOCIATED WITH THE LABOUR AND BIRTH

All women I speak to, and myself included have a level of fear associated with the actual labour and birth. I addressed my fears by doing hypnotherapy which takes you into a deep state of relaxation and really helps with anxiety and fear that many of us experience. I also read books on birth skills, and these practical skills combined with relaxing my mind helped me approach the baby's birth day feeling more confident. No one feels 100% confident with their first child birth experience, it is all about doing what you can to understand the process and then having a Midwife or Obstetrician you trust. There is no right and wrong and even the best birth plan, may not be able to be followed if complications arise - so never feel like a failure if your birth doesn't go to plan.

Join me on social media
with over 60k followers

www.livingbeautyfitness.com

INSTAGRAM
@livingbeautyamelia

FACEBOOK
Amelia Ricci Sports Model Fitness Trainer

YOU TUBE
Amelia Ricci 4 week bikini body health and fitness

NUTRITION FOR HEALTHY PREGNANCY

While pregnancy is an amazing time in your life and the greatest gift is your beautiful baby, it can also be challenging. The hormonal fluctuations, fatigue, increased appetite and changes in your body can lead to a rollercoaster of emotions. There is sometimes an overload of information and growing fear of eating unsafe foods and the worry of gaining too much weight.

So, where to start if you want to move forward, giving your body nourishment to grow, but also keeping yourself energised and heathy for the months that remain?

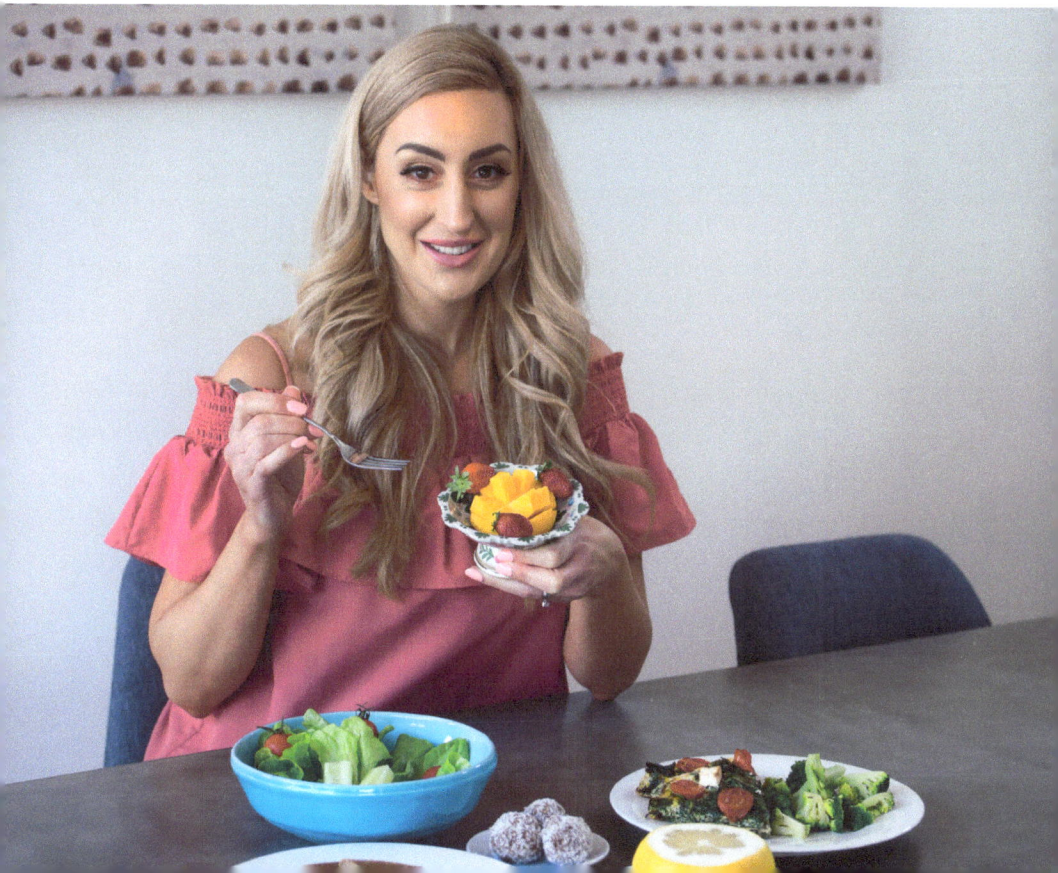

HOW MUCH WEIGHT SHOULD YOU GAIN DURING PREGNANCY?

There is a need to prepare yourself and accept that there will be weight changes and the worst thing you can do is get out your scale every day and check your weight. Scale weight includes the baby, fluid, placenta and your own muscle, skeletal structure and body fat. It is not useful to weigh yourself unless directed by a medical practitioner.

With many women feeling the need to return to pre-pregnancy weight almost instantly post-pregnancy, there is a growing concern of unrealistic weight goals during pregnancy.

Pre-Pregnancy BMI*	Total weight gain (kg)	Rates of weight gain in 2nd and 3rd Trimester (average gain per week)
Underweight (<18.5)	12.5 - 18	0.51kg
Normal (18.5 – 24.9)	11.5 - 16	0.42kg
Overweight (25 – 29.9)	7-11.5	0.28kg
Obese (>30)	5-9	0.22kg

*Institute of Medicine, weight gain during pregnancy, recommendations by pre-pregnancy BMI

The expected rate of weight gain is determined by the mother-to-be's pre-pregnancy BMI. Therefore, someone who was overweight would expect to gain a little less than someone who was underweight. Realistic expectations of weight gain, coupled with self-monitoring, support and education can reduce the risks assocted with excessive weight gain.

EATING THE RIGHT NUTRIENTS DURING PREGNANCY

You don't need to be on a strict plan. Eating healthily is making sure you get an appropriate amount of the essential nutrients for yourself and for the baby to grow. Pregnancy creates extra demands on a range of nutrients such as iron, folate and iodine. Most of these can be obtained through a balanced wholefoods diet and some also choose to take a pregnancy supplement such as Elevit or similar.

Protein

Protein is essential for cell growth and repair and commonly found in animal products, legumes and dairy based foods. As a rule, during the first trimester 0.8 grams of protein per kilo of body weight is required. This increased to one gram per kilo of body weight during the second and third trimesters.

Iron

The recommended intake of iron increases considerably to 27mg per day. The foods that contain iron are red meat, chicken and seafood, but also plant based sources such as beans and lentils, plus leafy greens. Absorption from plant-based sources can be enhanced by consuming them with vitamin C based foods such as broccoli, oranges, kiwi fruit and berries.

Folate

Folate is a B group vitamin commonly found in legumes, dark leafy greens, asparagus, broccoli, citrus and folate fortified foods. Folic acid supplementation of 400 micrograms is recommended.

Iodine

Iodine is important for the thyroid hormone, which is essential for growth and development. A supplement of 150 micrograms of iodine per day is recommended.

Calcium

There is no need for additional calcium other than the recommended 2.5 serves per day for women, many of us have however avoided or reduced dairy and moved to dairy free alternatives. It is important that we assess our calcium levels and consume adequate foods such as sardines, almonds and calcium fortified dairy free milks if following a low dairy diet.

Caffeine

As caffeine is known to cross the placenta and is a stimulant that has been linked to pre-term births and miscarriages, the American College of Obstetricians and Gynaecologists recommends that pregnant women should limit their intake to 200mg per day. A standard cappuccino gives you 155mg, instant coffee (1 tsp) provides 76mg, brewed coffee 137mg, brewed tea 48mg, Lipton tea 55mg, iced tea 48mg, red bull energy drink 80mg and V energy drink 109mg.

Suggestions to include	Foods to avoid
PROTEIN: Lean meat, chicken, fish, lentils, beans, tofu and cooked eggs. Canned tuna, salmon and sardines.	Deli meats.
IRON: Lean red meat, chicken, seafood, lentils, chick peas, dark leafy green vegetables	(Note: always try to prepare foods fresh where possible to avoid listeria)
CALCIUM: Dairy foods, sardines, almonds, calcium fortified non-dairy milks.	Soft cheese or surface ripened cheese such as brie or camembert

Dealing with Cravings:

* Trust your appetite, you can give into the crave but have a small amount and eat slowly and mindfully.

* Ensure you have protein and fibre at each meal as these nutrients can assist in controlling cravings.

* Plan your day and have your meals and snacks at hand for example raw almonds and some yoghurt and avoid skipping meals.

* Plan relaxation sessions where you rest to help reduce any stress you may be experiencing.

STAYING FIT DURING PREGNANCY
SAFE PREGNANCY EXERCISE GUIDE

Your body and mind will go through so many changes during pregnancy and it is important to understand the current guidelines on safe exercise during pregnancy, so you can follow guidelines and modify your routine accordingly. Active women experience less insomnia, stress, anxiety and depression and there is some evidence that exercise throughout pregnancy can reduce the length of labour. So, with all these great benefits it makes sense to stay active.

At the beginning of my first pregnancy I was terrified to exercise anything more than a gentle walk, as I had miscarried prior to conceiving my son Orlando. I blamed myself and wondered what I had done wrong, when in fact it was just Mother Nature's way of saying that this embryo was not the right one. So, during my first pregnancy, from 5 weeks I kept it simple and walked daily and did some gentle stretching and Pilates.

Throughout each trimester my confidence grew, and I was able to lift weights throughout the rest of my pregnancy and continue with light cardio exercise. It is important to realise that pre-exercise screening is important and that you work with a qualified exercise professional who cares for your needs individually, as there can be considerable variation between individuals and pregnancies. I did not overtrain, and I listened to my body with most sessions consisting of 20 minutes light cardio and 20 minutes of resistance training, followed by core and pelvic floor exercises and stretching.

Pregnancy and child birth have a major impact on a woman's body and every system is affected including respiratory, cardiac/circulatory, hormonal and musculoskeletal. The greatest changes experienced are usually postural, with an increased arch in the lower back and a rounding of the shoulders, lower back pain, separation of the abdominal muscles (Rectus Diastasis) and shortness of breath. I found that a positive attitude, sleeping longer at night, and taking breaks during exercise helped me get through my workouts.

Many women, including myself find the first trimester very challenging. This is where most of the cardiovascular changes occur and cardiac output is increased 30-50%, heart rate also increases 15%. I found this particularly hard when trying to do a light warm up with my personal training clients, I was out of breath and puffing – how embarrassing! Many women, including myself, also have morning sickness and/or all-day nausea.

In the second trimester, it's important to eliminate all ab workouts because as the stomach gets bigger, the risk of Rectus Diastasis increases with a tighter Rectus Abdominis. Not many people know this but your inner thigh muscles (adductors) attach to your public bone (pubic symphysis). As pregnancy advances the pubic bone starts to separate which can lead to pain. So, I always remove inner thigh work such as Pilates inner leg work or wide sumo squats as these can worsen the pain.

Finally, lying on your back (supine) is not recommended as many women feel nauseous or dizzy in this position. This is due to the weight of the baby pressing on the main blood vessels of the mother. One way to remedy this is to lie at a 45-degree angle for example if you wanted to keep doing a chest press movement, but at this stage (and in fact not from 14 weeks) no ab workouts from this time forward.

During pregnancy you always need to stay cool as the baby cannot regulate its body temperature, so ensure you remain hydrated and listen to the messages your body gives you. If something feels uncomfortable you need to stop and modify, and this is not a failure! You will recover so much faster post baby if you follow guidelines during your pregnancy rather than trying to do everything you did pre-pregnancy! This is not a time for PB's in the weights room, nor smashing yourself and reaching a peak heart rate. These days everyone wants to stay fit and lean, but I found that the greatest gift is a healthy baby and the more I keep this front of mind I don't care about the physical changes and am happy to train at a lower intensity. You have a lifetime to train hard!

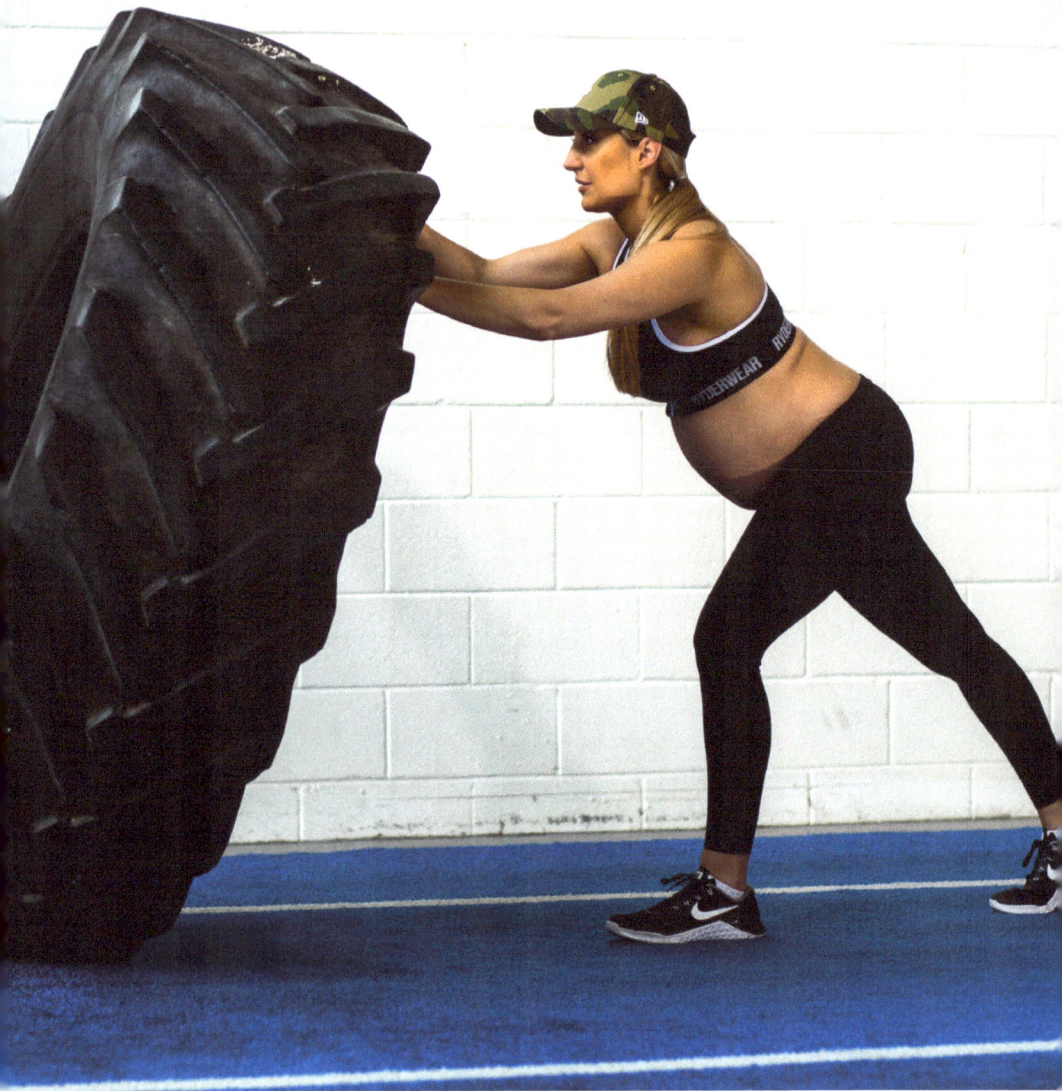

So, let's break it down and look at the stages of pregnancy and the guidelines from the latest published research and medical experts:

FIRST TRIMESTER
(WEEK 1 TO 12)

During the first trimester major physiological changes are taking place, even though you might not see much on the outside of your body. Blood volume expands, the uterus enlarges and during this time the foetus is undergoing its most important growth, including development of organs and limbs.

Past exercise history

Women who were exercising prior to their pregnancy may continue, but are advised to modify their exercise according to the physiological changes associated with their pregnancy. Women who were previously inactive need to start at a low level and progress gradually.

Intensity

Both aerobic and resistance training at moderate intensity are considered safe. Monitoring exercise intensity is important via both perceived exertion and heart rate measurement.

Duration and Frequency

It is recommended that the duration of the exercise session be limited to avoid hypoglycaemia and overheating. Increasing body temperature dramatically should be avoided, and if dehydration and high temperature are combined this can be detrimental to the developing baby.

SECOND TRIMESTER
(WEEK 13 TO 27)

One of the most important considerations in the second trimester is from 16 weeks, to avoid all exercises lying on your back because this can lead to vena cava compression (a major artery that delivers blood to your baby). Some other references suggest 20 weeks is the time to start avoiding laying supine, but I think the best approach is to be cautious. This took a bit of getting used to, however I soon found many alternatives such as using an incline bench for weights or side lying leg exercises on a mat.

This exciting trimester is where you will start to feel your baby move, almost like little flutters, or like a butterfly sensation in your stomach. You will feel your core muscles start to weaken or "turn off" as they make way for the changes your body is about to undergo, with regards to the structure of the abdominal wall. Don't worry or be scared, this part of pregnancy can mean low energy levels and you will need to get used to an altered centre of gravity, but everything is progressing nicely, making way for the growth of your beautiful baby.

At first when my abs started to relax, and my core was not as strong during functional movement, I found I had a lot of pain in my lower back as I struggled to adjust to this new posture. Walking relieved my back pain as did Pilates and stretching. Pilates exercises provide many benefits and allows women to achieve safe and healthy pregnancies by teaching postural muscle awareness and how to stabilise effectively during these great physiological changes.

Some of my favourite Pilates exercise included four-point balancing and then challenging stability by extending the opposite arm and leg, whilst keeping my core engaged. I also found wall squats using the fit ball were beneficial. You will see these exercises in the next section in my You Tube videos.

Pilates exercises were useful in establishing stability, so I could continue with light weights exercises for example for biceps, triceps, shoulders and back. I also did unweighted free standing squats in the second trimester, but found this impossible by the time I reached the third trimester, when I modified this exercise by incorporating wall squats with a fit ball.

Great musculoskeletal changes in the pregnant woman's body can raise the risk of injury during exercise and this not only includes posture and balance, but also hormonal changes which can mean increased joint laxity and hypermobility. Therefore, I made sure that I was extra careful when transitioning between different weights exercises, for example I took care when bending down to pick up a barbell or dumbbells, to avoid back strain. Also, when stretching after my workout I never went to my full range of mobility.

THIRD TRIMESTER
(WEEK 28 TO BIRTH, APPROX. 40)

In the third trimester it is time to slow down even more! It can be challenging to do less and rest more, but this is very important as the load on the musculoskeletal system is at its highest. I found that decreasing my pace on the treadmill and exercise bike was important, as was the decreased amount of weight I lifted during my weights routine.

In the third trimester water based activities are highly recommended as the weightlessness experienced whilst submerged in water can relieve pressure in joins and enable exercise without the gravity experienced on land. An important guideline is that when exercising in water the temperature should not exceed 32 degrees Celsius.

It is also important to monitor your response to exercise throughout all stages of pregnancy for any sign of vaginal bleeding, persistent pelvic pain, fatigue and regular contractions and consult your medical practitioner should any of these occur.

In the third trimester I experienced pelvic girdle pain (also known as pubic symphysis or sacro-iliac pain) as the muscles around the hip bones relaxed and other stabilising muscles strained and contracted to give my body stability to sit, walk and move. I consulted my obstetrician and physiotherapist and used strategies such as putting weight on both feet when standing up from a sitting position and avoided any unilateral (one leg or single sided) exercises.

OVERALL PREGNANCY EXERCISE GUIDELINES

Include the following activities	Avoid the following activities
Gradual warm up and cool down.	High impact or jerky movements.
Focus on strengthening pregnancy specific muscles such as pelvic floor, core and postural muscles.	Avoid feeling hot, exhausted or excessively sweaty.
Modified strength training.	Sudden changes of position or intensity.
Modified positions for supine (lying on your back) activities e.g. four-point kneeling, sitting on a fit ball and side lying.	Any exercise that involves breath holding.
Flexibility and stretching to be limited to a comfortable range of movement.	Any exercise that places significant load on the abdominals or pelvic floor including abdominal curls/sit ups, planks/hovers.
Relaxation such as meditation at the end of a yoga or body balance class.	Contact activities (to minimise falls and excessive blows to the abdominal region).
Low impact activities such as stationary bike, walking and cross trainer at a low to moderate intensity.	Any exercise that may exacerbate a pregnancy related condition.
Avoid the risk of overheating by exercising in a well-ventilated or air-conditioned environment.	Eight bearing activities beyond comfortable range of movement.

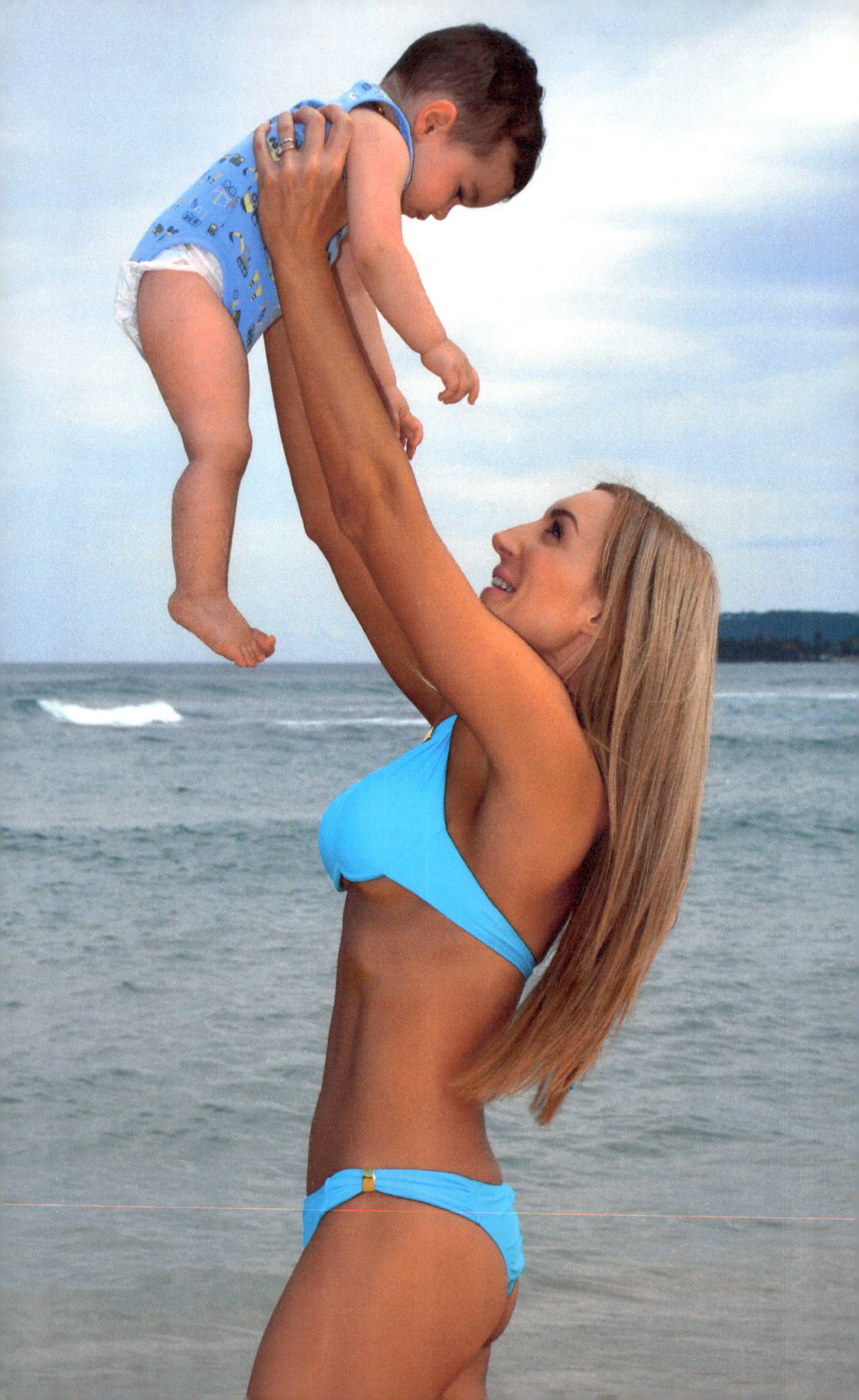

NUTRITION AND HYDRATION DURING EXERCISE
My experience during pregnancy

I found out the hard way not to get over hungry or too tired. If I did not rest each day, or went hours between meals, I would get extreme back pain and I would feel light headed and dizzy. Therefore, I always monitored the messages my body, and my baby were giving me. I looked at my macronutrient ratios and increased my carbohydrate intake and slightly decreased my protein, which made me to feel my best during pregnancy.

I recommend a small snack before and after exercise. A banana and a glass of low sugar coconut water gave me a good amount of energy and hydration during exercise. I also drank about 600ml of plain filtered water during every workout.

Post workout I would either go home to a nutritious meal of brown rice, stir fry vegetables and lean protein or if I was on the go, I made sure I had something in my cooler bag for example a plain organic yoghurt and a piece of fruit.

During my workout I made sure I positioned myself near an air-conditioner or fan if indoors or if exercising outdoors I would avoid the heat of the day and take morning walks whilst the weather was cool. As mentioned in the above guidelines, overheating can put your developing baby at risk. As a mum to be, you are likely to feel warmer throughout your pregnancy and therefore you want to reduce the heat whilst exercising, to avoid feeling faint or becoming dehydrated.

As I progressed to the later stages of my pregnancy with Orlando he was extremely active, which was a wonderful feeling. If he was moving a lot, I would stop exercising and take a few deep breaths. It is important to realise that stopping and resting mid cardio session or between weights sets is vital to listen to your body. I allowed myself to slow down and just enjoy the beautiful gift of growing a baby.

Take Home Messages

* Exercising during pregnancy requires modification and listening to your body, however it can be done safely.

* Pregnancy is not the time for achieving any personal bests, but rather using light weight training to retain your strength and stay active.

* Always bring water and pre- and post-workout snacks along to your workout, to give you and your baby hydration and nutrients. Fresh fruit is a good option because it is easily digested even when pressure on the digestive system is increased and you may not feel like eating much.

* Accept that you will need to reduce the intensity, duration and frequency of your workouts. If you feel tired have several rest days each week. Every trimester will be associated with varying levels of tiredness and rest should be prioritised over exercise.

* The benefits of exercise include a faster return to pre-pregnancy fitness and an increased ability to cope with the physical demands of motherhood.

* Pregnancy specific Pilates with a qualified practitioner or physiotherapist will do wonders for your weights and cardiovascular routine because it will assist you to maintain pelvic floor, core muscles and improve posture.

* All pregnant women are encouraged to work with their Obstetrician to discuss the appropriateness for their unique situation prior to starting or continuing any exercise routine and this may need to be reviewed and adapted during various stages of the pregnancy.

TRAINING IDEAS FOR YOUR PREGNANCY

Watch the You Tube videos at the links below to understand correct technique, modifications for pregnancy and see Amelia demonstrate the exercises whilst she is pregnant. The exercises below are suitable for both your home or gym workout. It is recommended you choose 5 exercises to start, perform 3 sets of 15 repetitions for each exercise with your total workout duration approximately 30 – 45 minutes and it's also very important to add a 10 minute stretch post workout and pelvic floor exercises.

3 Ways to make lunges more effective

(lunges with dumbbells)

Watch this video on You Tube: https://youtu.be/UKchdx92_OE

  a. Put 90% of your weight into your front heel

  b. Roll your knee outwards to feel the burn in your butt

  c. Sink lower so your thigh is parallel to the floor

Build a booty with weighted hip extensions

Watch this video on You Tube: https://youtu.be/MplhW9A0LEQ

  a. The medicine ball provides an unstable surface so your glutes and hamstrings need to work harder

  b. Add dumbbells for a challenge and/or place your feet on a medicine ball

  c. Keep your core tight and avoid rolling the hips to one side, keep them square

Best exercise for strong toned arms

Watch this video on You Tube: https://youtu.be/xyQsW3f5f-Q

a. Standing on one leg helps work your core

b. This is a great functional exercise

Legs and arms Blast

Watch this video on You Tube: https://youtu.be/vt7j6JFiJ-U

a. This looks easy but is advanced and challenges every muscle in your body

b. Try 10 reps each side without stopping

Work your triceps for insane arm tone

Watch this video on You Tube: https://youtu.be/Quky-_xSVjQ

a. Start with compound movements like bench dips

b. Follow with triceps extensions

c. Fully straighten your elbow every rep

5 simple pregnancy exercises for every trimester

Watch this video on You Tube: https://youtu.be/8_DD_1jrdXQ

a. Experts agree, when you're expecting, it's important to keep moving: Pregnant women who exercise have less back pain, more energy, a better body image and, post-delivery, a faster return to their pre-pregnancy shape. Being fit doesn't have to mean a big-time commitment or fancy equipment. The following workout is a recommendation, but it is important to consult your medical professional to be cleared for your specific circumstances during your unique pregnancy.

1. Wall squats
2. Bent over row (single arm)
3. Bicep Curls
4. Side lateral raises
5. Glute activation exercises with the resistance band

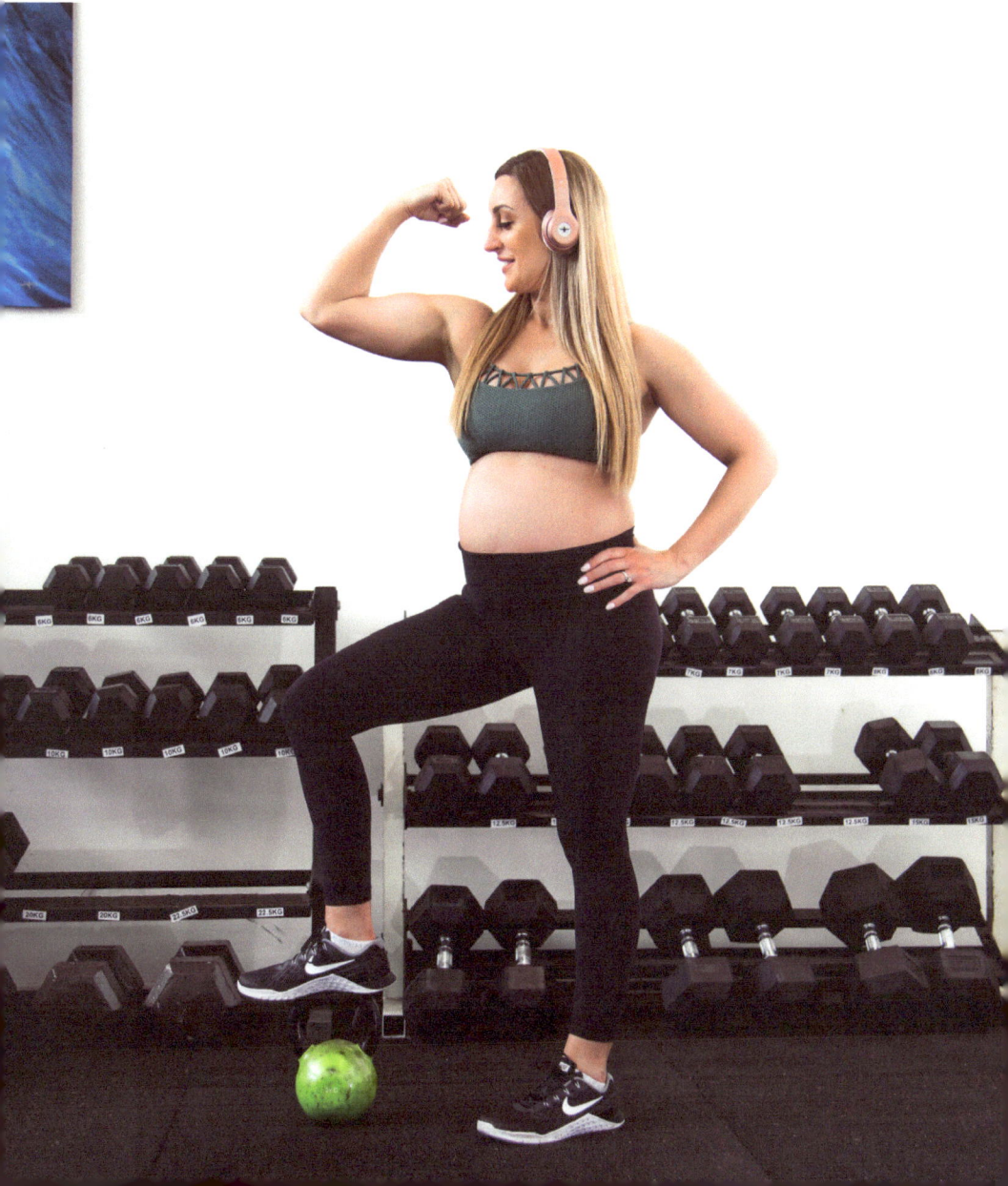

POST BABY SHAPE UP
PHASE 1 WORKOUT PROGRAM

This is such a special time to embrace your new bundle of joy, but it can also be very tiring as the lack of sleep and feeding schedule take much of your energy. I encourage you to take your time and be patient as your body needs time to heal. Most of all be kind to yourself with your expectations of how you look and set realistic goals for your exercise program.

Your body and mind go through so many changes during pregnancy and labour, so it's important to tailor a program to your needs and rebuild your strength slowly. This exercise program is a suggestion of what may suit you and it's important that you consult your medical practitioner prior to commencing and adjust exercises according to your unique situation.

A new baby brings joy and excitement to every family and it's essential to reflect on this great achievement of bringing new life into the world, and not pressure yourself to whip back into shape fast. It's vital you follow a gradual progression with specific exercises firstly focusing on rebuilding your deep abdominal muscles.

IMPORTANT CONSIDERATIONS FOR YOUR POST BABY EXERCISE PROGRAM

What type of birth did you have?

Caesarean births require a surgical cutting of the abdominals which makes these muscles weaker than normal. The rehabilitation of the core muscles takes time and in the early stages you need to follow exercises prescribed by a specialist physiotherapist. Care must also be taken when returning to exercise and it's suggested you follow a gradual progression of exercise intensity.

Did you have any complications such as pelvic floor issues or abdominal separation?

You might think it's okay start where you left off pre-baby, but there have been so many changes in your body that this could worsen abdominal separation or cause further weakening of your pelvic floor muscles.

Monitoring exercise intensity is important and if any pain is experienced you should rest. Care must be taken with heavy weight training and starting with lighter weights is recommended. Running or jumping exercises are to be avoided.

It is recommended that the duration of your exercise session be monitored and build up slowly each week rather than trying to return to a full workout.

Have you experienced any pain since your labour and what movements cause this pain?

It's a busy time when you return from the hospital and start the routine of being a mother, so take some time to observe your daily movements and consider whether you have any specific weaknesses for example in bending forward over the cot to pick up your baby, leaning over to put your baby in the car, or in daily activities such as carrying groceries. If you have back pain, hip pain or abdominal pain it's important that you undertake rehabilitation exercises prior to commencing any exercise program.

What is your past exercise history?

Women who were exercising throughout their pregnancy will normally be able to return to their program within a few months, but are advised to modify their exercise according to the physiological changes associated with their labour. Women who were previously inactive need to start at a low level and progress gradually.

What is the best way to get flat abs post baby?

Crunches are not the most effective exercise to flatten the abdominals because they work the superficial layers (the rectus abdominis). To achieve flat abs, you need to work the deep layers of abdominal muscles that will support your posture, narrow your waist and increase stamina during a busy day caring for bubs. Focusing on core strength, these exercises combine stretching and strengthening, with breathing and coordination to create a balanced body.

What are the muscles used?

The most important muscles to achieve flat abs are the transversus abdominis. These muscles act as a corset and wrap around the torso from the front to the back of the body. The transversus abdominis is the deepest layer of the abdominal muscles and is also a stabiliser of the spine. This muscle is the most important of all the abdominal muscles because these postural muscles support the body through the rigours of everyday life.

The other core stabilising muscles targeted in this exercise guide, are the pelvic floor, gluteal muscles and multifidus. The exercises in this guide also strengthen the internal and external obliques.

So, now that we understand everyone is different and progression to a full exercise program should be gradual, let's look at some simple and effective exercises for your post baby shape up.

PHASE 1
(FROM 6 TO 20 WEEKS POSTPARTUM)

Working on the activation of your deep abdominal muscles is an important foundation for your post baby workout. In addition to walking, this exercise program may be suitable for you from 6 weeks post birth. **Always get clearance from your medical practitioner.

Not sure how to activate the transversus abdominis?

Watch the video here on You Tube: https://www.youtube.com/watch?v=v-8v7yJu6IU

Towel squeeze

Lie on your back with a large towel rolled and placed between your knees. Take a deep breath in and as you breathe out draw your navel towards your spine and squeeze the towel between your knees. Hold for 10 seconds and repeat 3 times, with a break to rest in between.

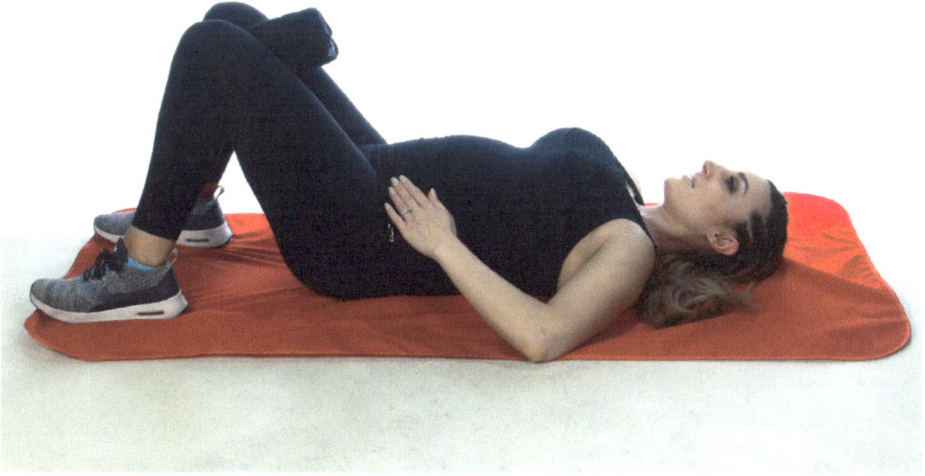

Leg slides

Lie on your back with your fingers placed just inside your hip bones. Take a deep breath in and as you breathe out draw your navel towards your spine and slide one leg out along the floor trying to keep your pelvis still and the return to the start position. Repeat 4 times alternating sides, rest and repeat.

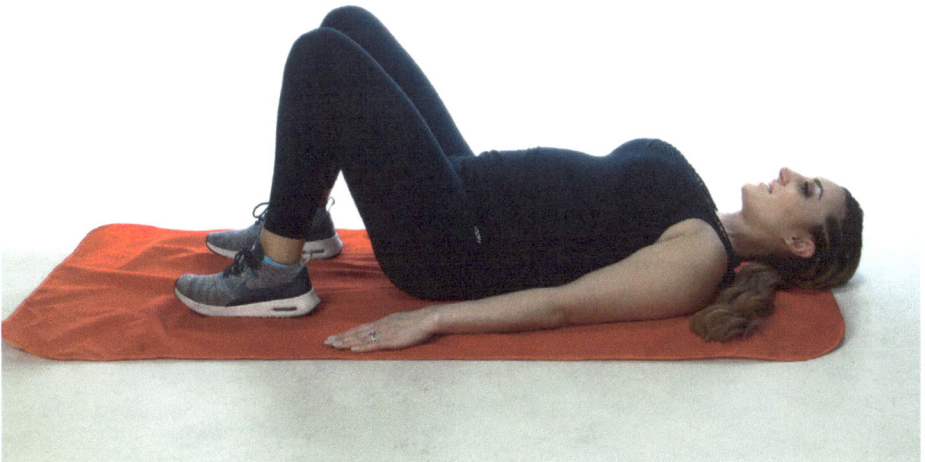

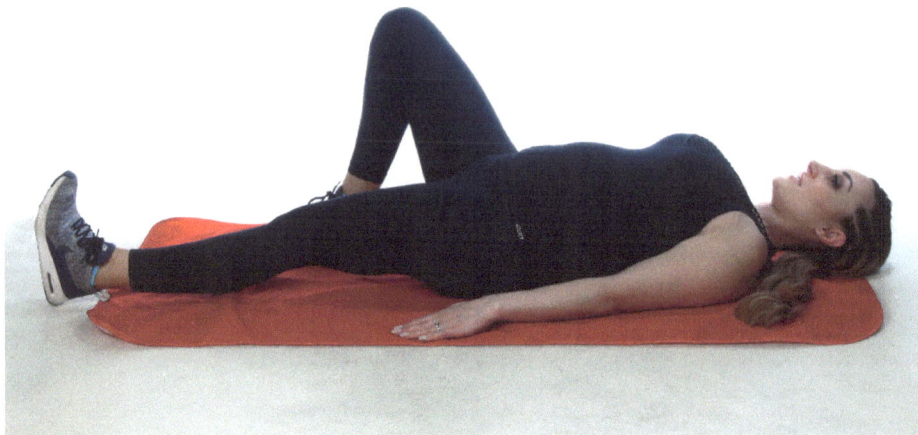

Single leg extension

Lie on your back with your hands at your sides. Raise your hips up into a pelvic curl position squeezing your butt and drawing your navel to your spine. If you feel strong enough you can begin to slowly extend one leg out, keeping your thighs parallel. Progress this exercise by keeping the hips lifted and performing 8-10 repetitions in total, then rest and repeat.

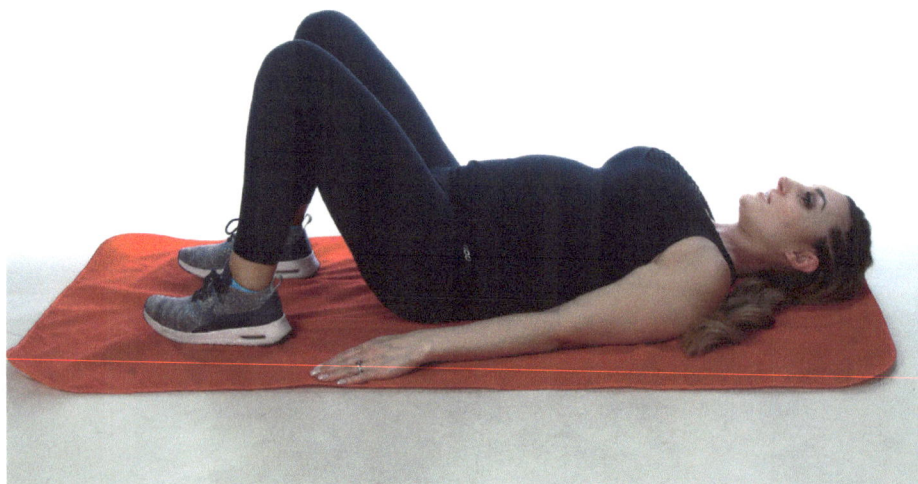

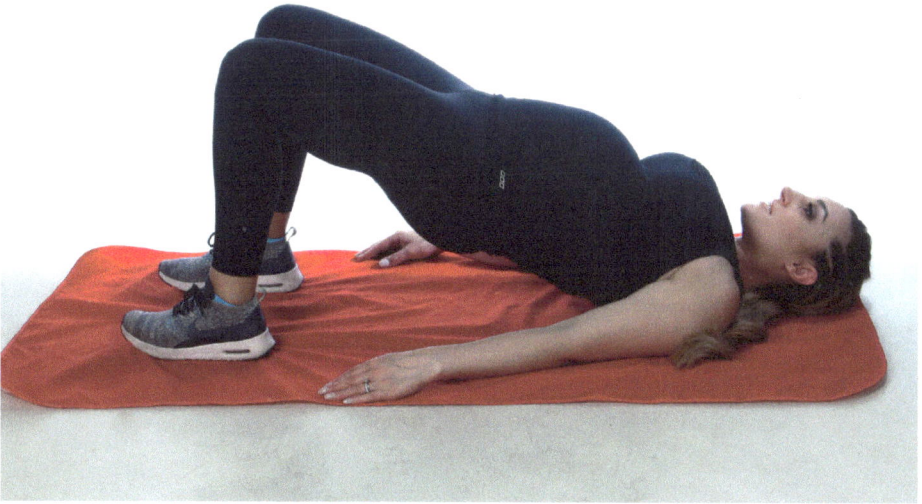

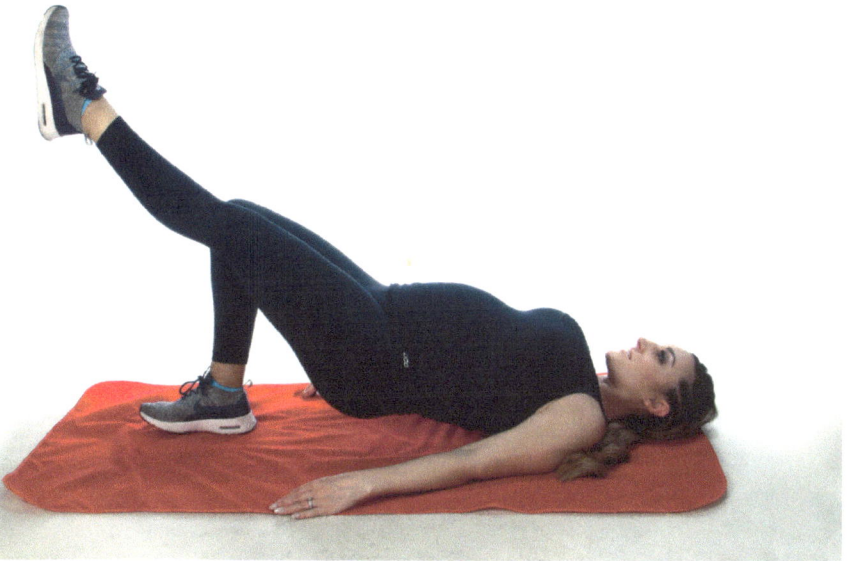

Resistance band back work

Stand with your feet hip distance apart, engage your abs by drawing your navel tight as if you are tightening a belt around your waist. Squeeze your shoulder blades together and hold for a second then release. Perform 3 sets of 10 reps.

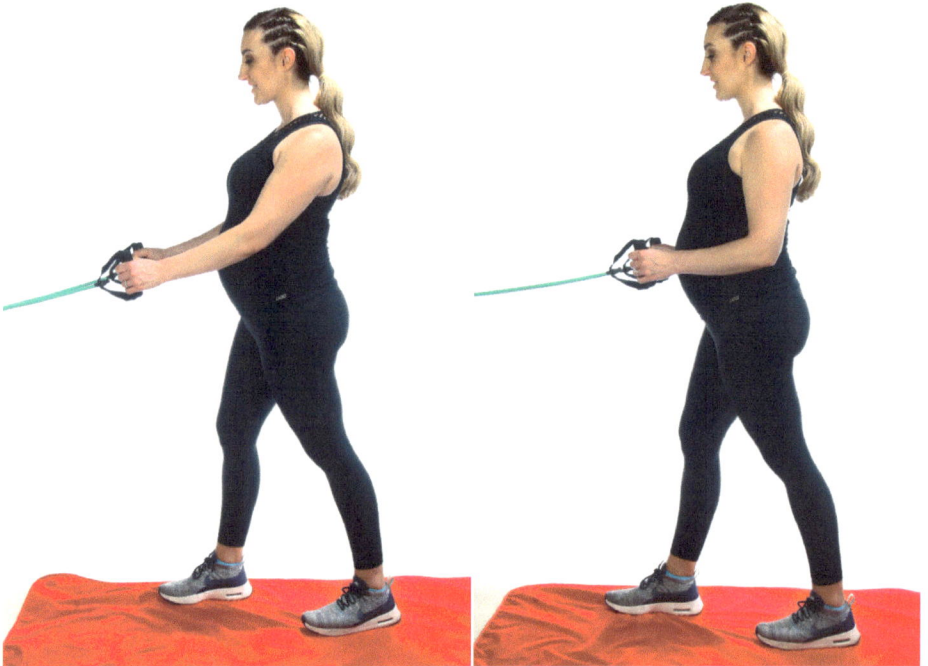

Clam position

Lie on your side with your arm extended, knees bent and feet back in line with your hips. Keep your deep abs engaged as you squeeze your heels together and raise your top knee upwards using the butt to initiate the movement. Perform 15 reps each side and 3 sets in total, resting in between sets or when you need to.

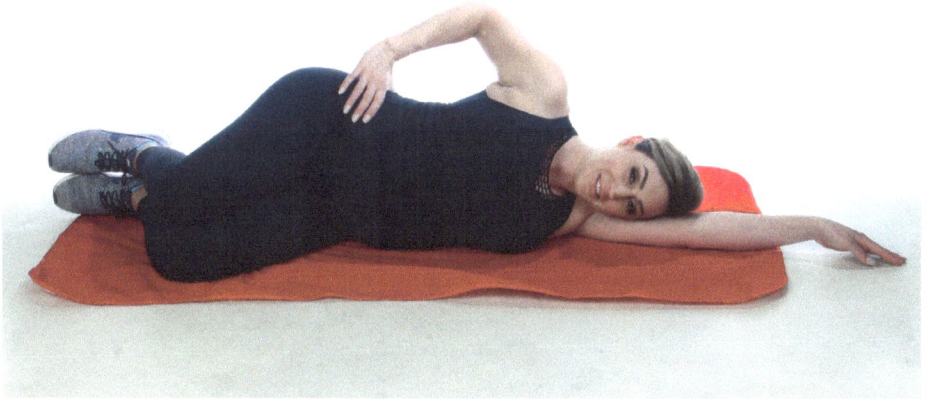

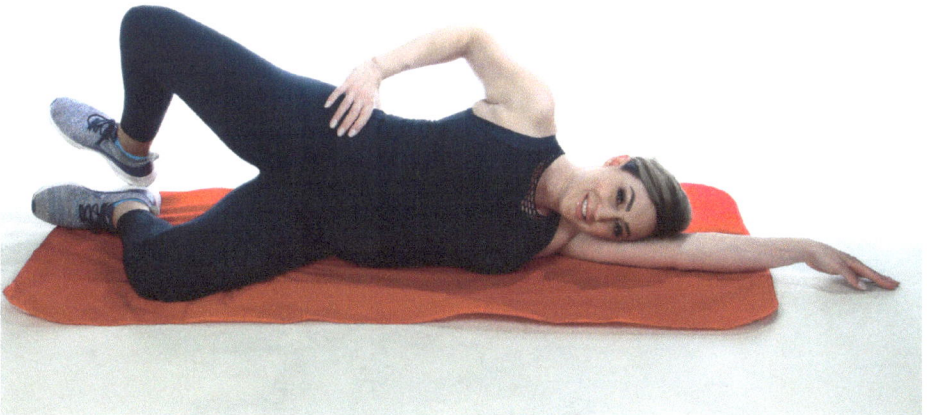

Opposite arm and leg extension

The all fours opposite arm & leg extension has two parts. Firstly, you should work on extending just your legs:

Part 1

Start on your hands and knees. Slowly extend one leg straight out behind you. Hold 3-5 seconds. Slowly bring your leg back down and repeat with the opposite leg, again holding 3-5 seconds. Repeat 5-10 times on each side.

Part 2

When you can extend your legs with ease, you can add the arms: Slowly extend your right leg and your left arm. Hold 3-5 seconds. Slowly bring your leg and arm back down and repeat with your left leg and right arm, again holding 3-5 seconds. Repeat 5-10 times on each side.

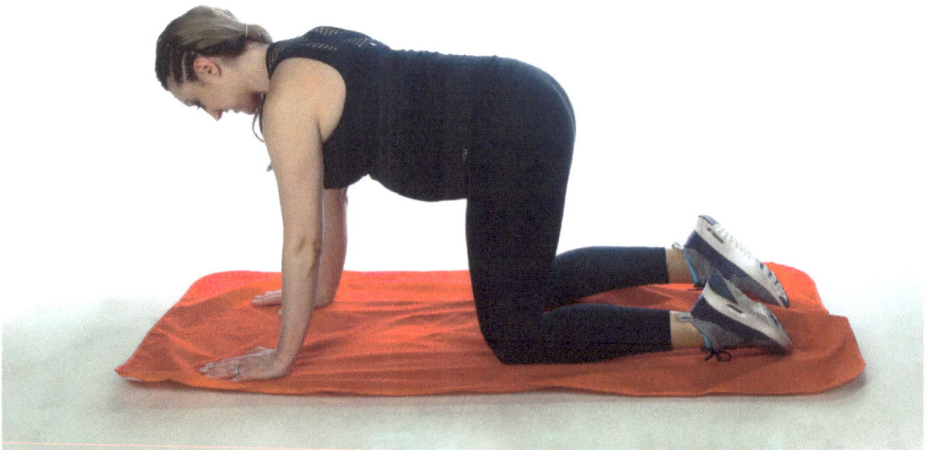

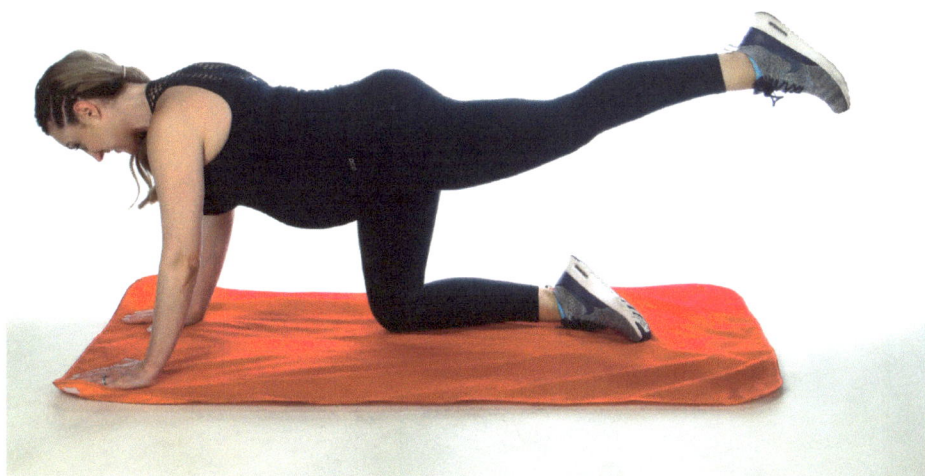

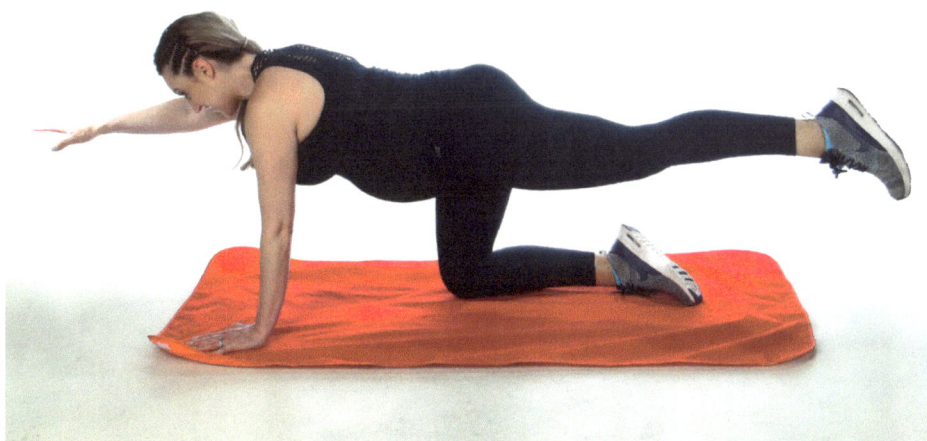

PHASE 2
(FROM 12 WEEKS POSTPARTUM ONWARDS)

Building on the foundation of postural strength you can now add light dumbbells and progress to full body movements. Monitor how your body is feeling and modify the exercises by performing them without weights to begin and slowly progress over several weeks. This is where you can move onto the Original 4-week Bikini Body Program. This may be from 12 weeks postpartum onwards.

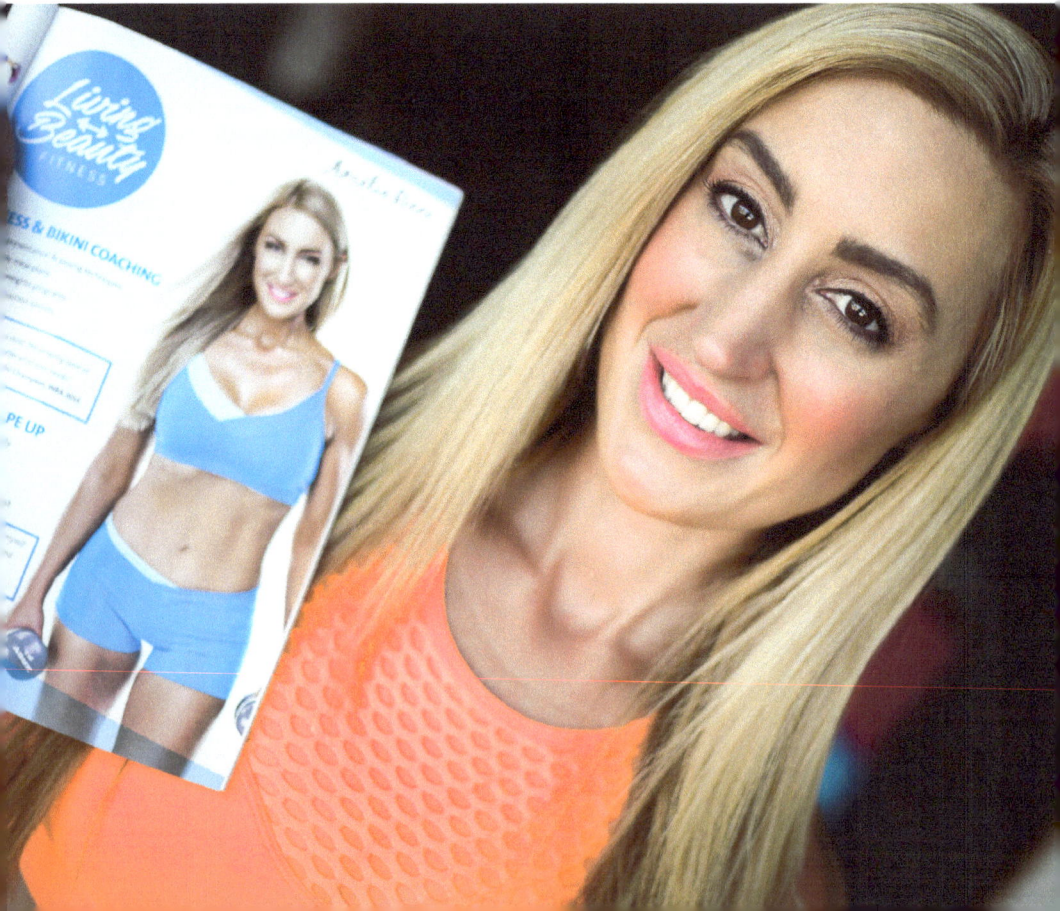

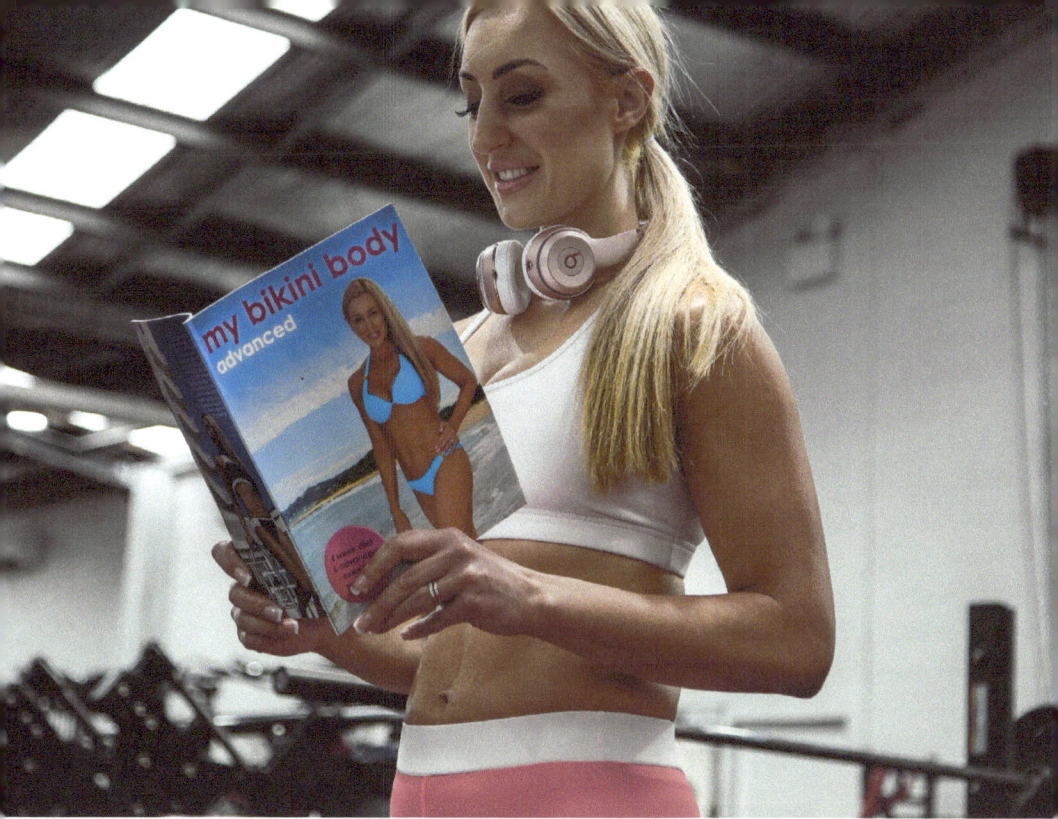

PHASE 3
(FROM 20 WEEKS POSTPARTUM ONWARDS)

In phase 3 if you have done all the important internal work to rehabilitate pelvic floor and maintained consistency with your weight training you will be ready for your next challenge. The 4 week Bikini Body Advanced program is your next step.

These programs give you the exact meal plans, training routines and motivation tips that Amelia used to lose 25KG after her first pregnancy and also helped hundreds of women lose weight and tone up their body.

5 ESSENTIAL TIPS FOR LOSING THE BABY WEIGHT:

1) Consistency

If you miss a day of exercise or fall off the wagon with your meal plan it is ok, you are human. The key to success is consistency over time.

2) Goal Setting

Set a goal for example 4 weeks and do your measurements weekly during this time. Then re-set your goal for another achievable time period.

3) It is OK to spend time on you

Being a mum is the most rewarding role ever and you love your bub so much it is hard to avoid feeling guilty for spending time away from them. However you will feel refreshed and stronger from regular exercise and your baby will benefit from having a mum who has so much more energy to play and laugh with them.

4) Incorporate weights and resistance training

Weights are key to changing the shape of your body and by incorporating light weights to begin with, this can be done safely and effectively to sculpt your legs, butt and abs back into shape.

5) When to move onto a more challenging fitness program?

Each of the programs suggested in this exercise guide need to be followed with consistency and when you have established a routine you will be able to tell if you can move on to the more advanced program, or continue with the current program for an extended duration. It is always best to follow a program with perfect technique, performing the exact sets and reps before moving onto the next stage.

Following a gradual progression for your post baby exercise program will ensure you engage the deep ab muscles and build core strength as the foundation for long term strength and reduce the risk of injuries by rushing back into your normal program too soon.

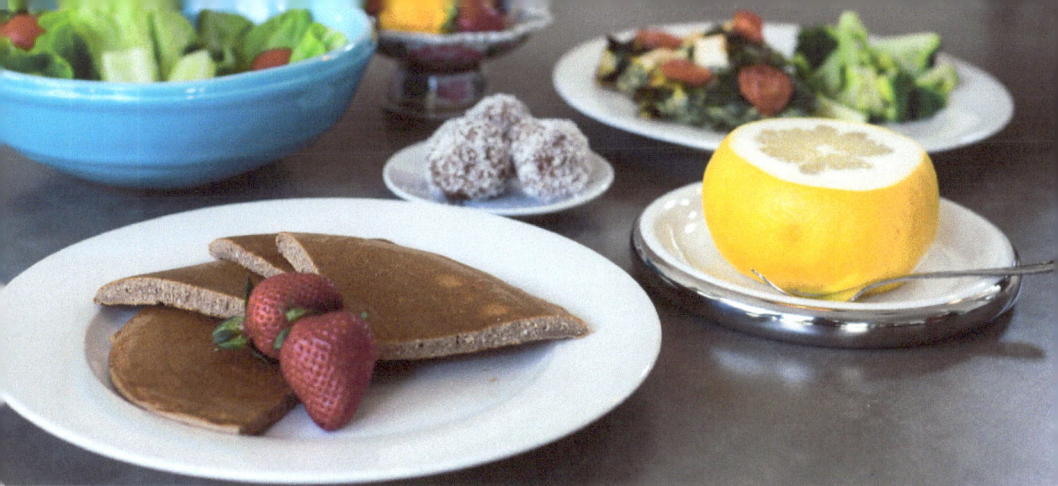

POST BABY MEAL IDEAS TO NOURISH MOTHER AND BABY

As a new mum it is easy to fall into the trap of drinking numerous cups of coffee and eating comfort food every day. With sleep deprivation and little time to think about yourself, one day can pass so quickly and then you realise its dinner time and you may not have had a healthy meal.

Even as a fitness professional (who should know better) I have been there! However, these poor food choices made me feel terrible and did nothing for my health and fitness goals.

If your baby is six months of age it is time to introduce solids. This can be daunting to try and think of healthy snacks to compliment milk feeds. This article provides ideas (based on literature from Australian and world health organisations) that can be adapted for your own snacks, so that you can eat at the same time as your baby or toddler. This will help you make nourishing food choices and give you more energy to cope with the demands of being a mum.

Baby and toddler foods matched with my favourite 'go to' snacks for mums and bubs on the go.

Food	Baby or toddler's snack	Fit mums snack
Wholegrain rolled oats cooked with water.	Puree or mash with steamed pears.	Add chocolate WPI (whey protein isolate) protein powder and walnuts to make porridge.
Sweet potato, steamed or boiled.	Mash with avocado.	Serve with chicken breast fillet and hummus.
Chicken Breast fillets roasted in the oven with lemon juice and parsley.	Puree or chop finely and combine in the blender with a can of drained chick peas for a creamy texture. Older toddlers can eat raw or steamed carrot sticks and use the mixture as a dip.	Serve with brown rice, broccoli and snow peas or make a chicken sandwich with salad.
Plain yoghurt (no added sugar).	Finely chop strawberries and mash into the yoghurt.	Combine yoghurt with blueberries and almonds.
Raw carrot and cucumber.	Grate carrot and cucumber and mix with ricotta cheese for a smooth texture.	Dip raw sticks or carrot and cucumber into a low-fat tzatziki dip.
Chia seeds soaked in water.	Mix with banana and yoghurt.	Make a protein shake with water, vanilla WPI, cinnamon and banana. Blend with ice.

Oven roasted pumpkin, cubed.	Puree or mash with steamed baby spinach.	Add chunks of pumpkin to a fry pan with ½ cup of egg whites from a carton and top with sliced tomato to make an omelette.
Salmon pieces (skinless and boneless) baked or steamed with fresh coriander and lemon.	Puree with steamed zucchini.	Serve fish fillets whole with steamed zucchini and a dollop of sour cream for flavour.
Hard boiled eggs.	Mash with avocado and grated cheese or serve cut in half as a finger food.	Serve hard boiled eggs with a handful of raw almonds and celery or cucumber sticks.

WHAT SHOULD TODDLERS AND BABIES EAT?

The department of Health in Australia recommends that a variety of nutritious foods be incorporated daily and these include: vegetables, fruit, dairy foods, lean meat, breads, cereals, rice and pasta. Their guidelines also state that salt and sugar should not be added to foods.

It is also important to consider allergies when introducing new foods. Therefore, when introducing new foods to your baby, follow the 3-day rule: only one new food every three days to target the source of any potential allergic reaction. Remember always consult with your child's paediatrician before introducing solid foods to your baby and specifically discuss any foods that may pose allergy risks for your child.

Recommended drinks

Babies and toddlers will vary with the amount of milk they drink, and this may include breastfeeds or formula. Plain tap water is also recommended by health organisations and is said to be the best drink as it is cost effective and prevents tooth decay.

Tips for healthy and happy meal times

* Toddlers need to eat small amounts often. The guideline is 3 small meals and 2-3 snacks.

* Sit down together and relax, whether it be at a café, park or at home. Give meals and snacks plenty of time.

* Eat together so your child can see the family eating a wide range of foods.

* Be patient and do not worry or dismiss a certain food if your child does not immediately like it, or makes a funny face! They will take time to get used to new textures and flavours.

* If you provide healthy food, your child will decide to eat the amount they choose, try to avoid battling about the amount they eat. Let their appetite guide how much they eat.

* As a mum never feel guilty about taking time to eat your meals and drink water. It is important that you are fit and healthy as you will have greater energy to care for your little one.

* Make some meals ahead of time that freeze well so you are never stuck without a meal.

10 BEST TIME SAVINGS TIPS FOR FIT MUMS

Before you became a mum, you could go to the gym every day, have a sleep in on Sunday's and spend time catching up with friends over coffee at your leisure. But this all changes when you have a little one who depends on you for their every need.

Schedules can be unpredictable and there are days when time escapes you and before you know it, the clock says 9pm, and you're still doing loads of washing!

Don't give up if you have days where you are in tears and struggling to cope. On my journey as a new mum, I have learned that this is completely normal and just because I have a bad day, tomorrow will be better.

Whether you have one child or five, all mothers work incredibly hard to balance the around this challenging around-the-clock job. And, because the job does not give you days off, there is no time to catch up. Not only will these tips give you more time, you will feel happier because you can accomplish the health and fitness goals that are important to you.

1. CHANGE YOUR PACE

Slow down a little and delegate where you can. Cut down your own 'to do' list so others can help with the workload. It can be hard to accept offers of help from friends and family, but this will allow you to schedule some time for yourself, including your fitness goals.

2. FOCUS ON ONE GOAL EACH WEEK

Getting things done can be as simple as giving yourself ONE main thing to focus on each week. If you choose your focus each week, for example starting a new weights program, or stretching your muscles before bed at night, this will ensure your wellbeing. The same applies for looking after your family, for example organising your child's school books ahead of time, or for younger children starting a new activity that helps their development.

Small steps towards your fitness goals really add up, especially when you look back over the year. And, when we look at our children they also thrive when given small steps towards their learning and growth.

When broken down into smaller weekly actions, bigger goals always seem much more achievable and you will surprise yourself when you look back at the end of the year at what you have accomplished.

3. STOP WASTING TIME

How much time do you spend in the digital world as compared to the real world? This applies to social media, television, mindless internet surfing and any other activity that involves staring at a screen.

Nature is so amazing. Why spend so many hours of your life staring at a screen or a computer? Get outdoors and spend quality time with your family, just having fun and being in the moment.

I know that I feel much more enriched by going to the beach or the park, than time spent at the computer or watching TV. Switch it off or set yourself time limits.

Audit your life and eliminate these time-wasting activities.

4. SAYING NO MEANS MORE TIME FOR YOU

You are being unfair to yourself by saying 'yes' to every request and commitment. Stay focused on what you want to achieve and simplify your life. You will feel less stressed and be more present in all situations.

Remember saying 'no' to others more often can mean saying 'yes' to yourself and doing things that make you happy.

5. PREPARATION IS KEY

Whether it is packing your gym bag the night before or preparing your meals in advance, preparation and organisation are key.

Prepare all your meals in advance, but on the weekend, do some extra cooking and freeze portions. I find that if I do not prepare my meals in advance, time escapes me during my busy week and I am more likely to make unhealthy choices that do not meet my fitness goals.

I cook several kilos of protein at one time and I freeze these portions. I will also bake vegetables, and these are great to puree for baby food. It is so much easier to eat a healthy diet when you can feed the same foods to your children.

6. STAY ORGANISED AND HAVE A BASIC ROUTINE

Having an organised household can be unrealistic, but I am not talking about the daily mess of toys, bottles and laundry strewn around the house. Organising the items, you use daily can a lot of save time. For example, I sorted out which of my child's clothes still fit and stored away the outfits that are too small. This saves time when trying to get ready in the morning.

Routine creates structure, and this leads to success. Even a basic routine, focusing on nap times, can be beneficial, despite the fact that it cannot always be adhered to. Having a basic routine that gives us the things we need each day will lead to ultimate wellbeing for the whole family.

7. PLAY AND FITNESS GO HAND IN HAND

Nothing lights up children's hearts more than adults playing with them. Play times can be outdoors and indoors and it is during these times that there is plenty of opportunity to combine fitness into your day together.

Walking to the park (if you have a baby) or using the play equipment with your children (if they are older) is not only fun, but it does not feel like exercise. Before you know it, you have had a great workout and your child or baby is probably ready for their next nap!

It saves so much time if you can combine spending time with your family and fitness activities that are enjoyable for everyone.

8. WORK BACK AND HOUR FROM WHEN YOU MUST LEAVE HOME

Aim to start getting your belongings together for an outing one hour before. That way you have everything ready when you must leave. It is much easier to leave the house when you gather everything you need together, ahead of time.

Pack your gym bag ahead of time and keep it in your car. Have your sneakers and gym clothing always packed and put this in the boot of your car straight away. You also might be able to fit in another workout unexpectedly.

9. KEEP A DIARY AND LISTS

Keeping a diary and writing lists, are great tools to manage your time, prioritising what is most important to you.

Children are so unpredictable which means being flexible is important, but having a plan in your diary gives you direction. So, if your day does not go according to plan, you will find a way to look back at your diary and your lists and re-schedule what is important to get done.

10. BELIEVE IN YOURSELF

Others in your life may not value their health and fitness, but this should not influence your choices.

Invest in your priorities and not only will you be happier, you will feel more in control of your time. Therefore, when it comes to spending time doing other household work that you don't enjoy, you will be more accepting because you have devoted some time to the things you do enjoy and value.

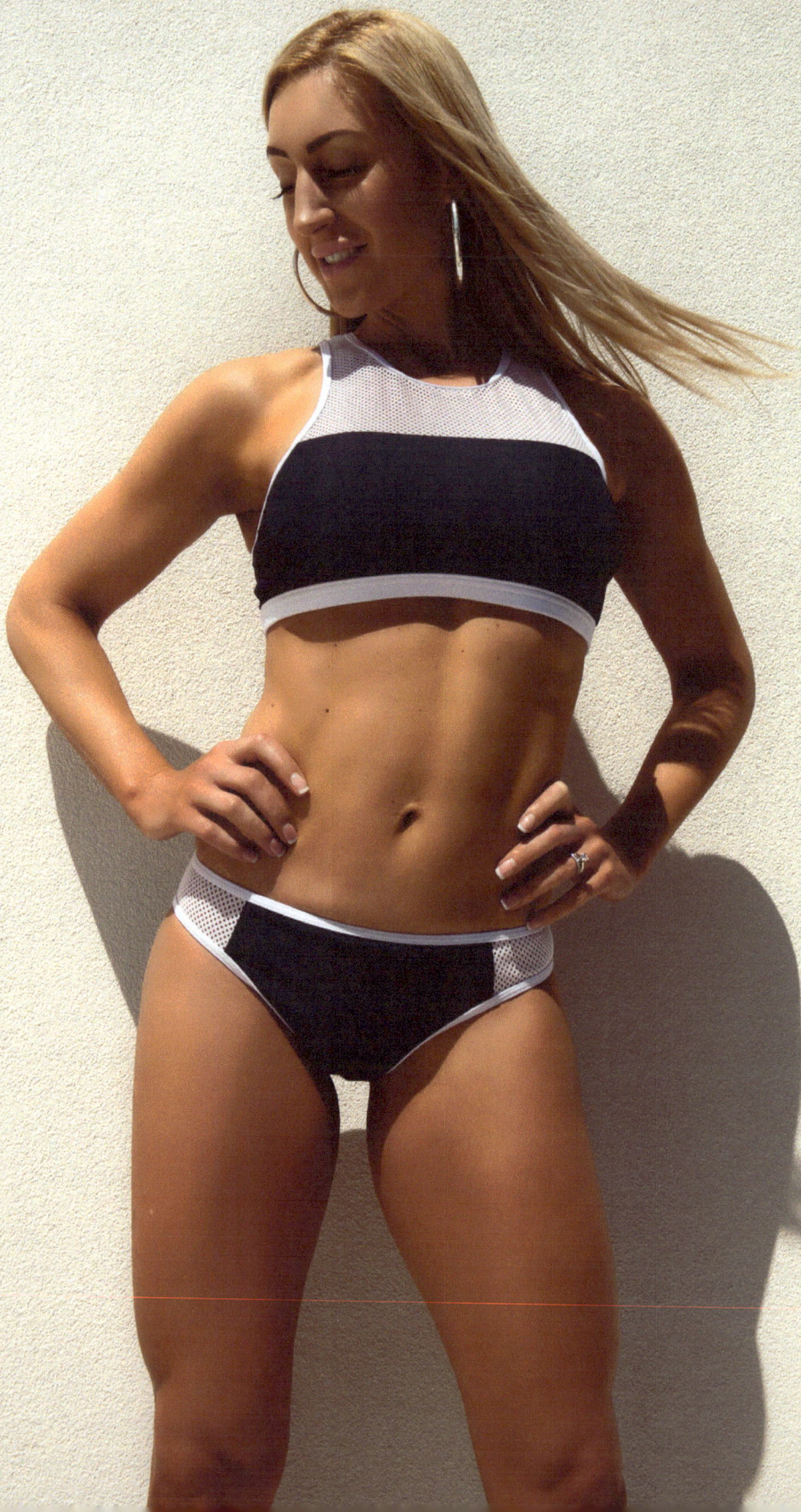

TAKE HOME MESSAGES

Accept you won't be able to achieve everything according to strict timelines. Be realistic with the time frames you set yourself for work projects or tasks at home.

Give yourself time to build up your strength and fitness. Don't read gossip magazines that show new mum's springing back to their pre-baby body within weeks, this is not realistic.

If you occasionally break down in tears and struggle to cope, don't feel like a failure, this is completely normal! Every mum has her breaking point and it is perfectly to fine to cry and let out your emotions. Being a mum is hard and every mother feels this way at some point.

And, finally avoid the super-woman mentality. Strive for balance to give yourself some time alone. This means accepting offers from friends or family who want to help you and don't try to do everything yourself.

STAY CONNECTED WITH AMELIA ON YOUR FITNESS JOURNEY

Amelia Ricci is a well-known Australian fitness model. Thanks to her balanced physique and years of weight training she has been featured in fitness magazines, commercials and loves creating workout videos. As a certified Fitness Expert and Pilates and Yoga trainer she helped thousands to transform their body. With 4WEEKBIKINIBODY she developed a 30-day transformation program which is based on 20 years' experience as a fitness model and coach.

Amelia believes perfection is boring and the way to feel great is to eat fresh clean foods, train hard, love yourself and never stop learning.

As a 2 x Fitness Model Champion and mentor to Australia's successful fitness and bikini models Amelia enjoys working in her business Living Beauty. Amelia has a series of four other eBooks which contains all her health and fitness principles at

www.livingbeautyfitness.com

You Tube: Amelia Ricci 4 week bikini body fitness
Facebook: AmeliaRicciSportsModelFitnessTrainer
Instagram: @livingbeautyamelia

REFERENCES

1. For further guidance contact your medical professional and a Registered Dietician at the link below:

   https://daa.asn.au/smart-eating-for-you/smart-eating-fast-facts/pregnancy/nutrition-for-pregnancy/

2. Edmonds, D, Dr Furness, D and Westlake, L (2013). Pre-and Post-Natal Exercise Guidelines. Fitness Australia.

3. Norton K & Norton, L (2011) Pre-Exercise Screening, Guide to the Australian adult pre-exercise screening system.

4. Bell, Dr BB, Dodey, Dr MM, (2009) Royal College of Obstetricians and Gynaecologists (RCOG Statement 4).

5. Artal, R, Clapp, J, Vigil, D (2014) American College of Sports Medicine.

6. Sports Medicine Australia Fact sheet,

   www.sma.org.au

7. Dene, L (2007), Pilates During Pregnancy, Network for Fitness Professionals.

8. Vladutiu, Dr C (2010), Physical activity and injuries during pregnancy, Journal of Physical Activity and Health, volume 7.

9. Brad A. Roy, Ph.D., FACSM, FACHE, Post-Partum Exercise (2014) American College of Sports Medicine.

10. Guiding principles for feeding non-breastfed children 6-24 months of age (2005) World Health Organization.

11. Start them right – A Parent's guide to healthy eating for under 5's (2008) Department of Health and Human Services, Tasmania.

12. Healthy Meals for Babies & Toddlers (2008) by Valerie Barrett.

Important: This wellness and exercise program is designed to promote health, fitness and a sustainable lifestyle. The information contained in this program is designed to be a guideline only. It is general information and is not intended to be specifically tailored to individual needs. Nor is this guide intended to be a substitute for professional medical advice, diagnosis or treatment. It is not formulated to suit any specific nutrient deficiencies, allergies or any other food or health-related problems. If you have, or suspect that you have, any of these issues, please seek the help of a medical professional for a fully tailored solution for you and your needs. You should use your own judgement and combine this with the advice from your medical professional.

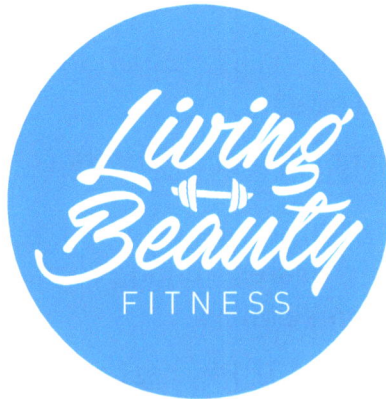

www.livingbeautyfitness.com

www.ingramcontent.com/pod-product-compliance
Lightning Source LLC
Chambersburg PA
CBHW041225280326
41928CB00045B/66